Sex Education for Toddlers to Young Adults

James Kenny

SEX EDUCATION
FOR TODDLERS
TO YOUNG ADULTS

A Guide for Parents

Nihil Obstat: Rev. Nicholas Lohkamp, O.F.M.
Rev. Christopher R. Armstrong

Imprimi Potest: Rev. Jeremy Harrington, O.F.M.
Provincial

Imprimatur: +James H. Garland, V.G.
Archdiocese of Cincinnati
December 13, 1988

The *nihil obstat* and *imprimatur* are a declaration that a book is considered to be free from doctrinal or moral error. It is not implied that those who have granted the *nihil obstat* and *imprimatur* agree with the contents, opinions or statements expressed.

Cover and book design by Julie Lonneman

ISBN 0-86716-110-8

Contents

Introduction

No other topic generates so much talk with so little information as does sex. Some people giggle and smirk at double meanings. Others are crude and gross in their sexual references. Few people talk about sex practically and sensibly and reverently.

In an education in any other area one would expect to learn about the nature of the subject, how wise and worthwhile it is and how to do it well. For example, if a woman needed to learn about her coming childbirth, no one would tell her not to take drugs during her pregnancy and not to smoke and then try to pass that off as a complete education in childbirth. A few negative warnings do not constitute a complete education.

Yet that unfortunately is what we often do in sex education. We give a few warnings about the misuse of sex, perhaps tell a few jokes about it, but say very little of practical worth. Sexual beginners are left to work out matters "in the dark."

This book attempts to remedy that situation, to go beyond the don'ts, to speak reverently of the mystery and beauty of genital sex, and most of all, to outline for parents how and when to offer a proper education in the physical aspects of sex.

Silence too long has been passed off as virtue. There are some plain facts which need to be stated simply and with reverence. There is a beautiful story here which needs to be told.

That story is, of course, much larger than the plain facts about physical sexual activity. But it is teaching the facts which parents have trouble doing; it is the effort to teach the facts that this book is intended to aid.

Chapter One

The Right Stuff

God, having chosen to visit the world, did not come as a VIP or a world leader or a minister of religion, but as a small baby into a family. When Jesus wanted to describe God, to tell us what God was like, how to imagine the Infinite, he used family names and roles. He spoke of God as his Father and himself as Son. One might gather from this that family is central to God's plan for sharing creative activity, perhaps even God's favorite invention.

The intimacy of marriage is most compellingly communicated through sex. Intercourse is *the* act special to marriage. More than that, sex has many wonderful faces, intricately woven together.

The Importance of Sex

Sex is the original Xerox machine, the way the human race copies and reproduces itself. Better than a Xerox because, as genetic information is actually exchanged and combined, sex offers the possibility for the human race to continue to improve itself through evolution.

From this exchange of genetic information, new and unique human beings are created. Because sex is the means by which people generate life, it is very *important*, perhaps the most important natural act a person can perform. Without sex, the race would die. No wonder a sense of awe and reverence surrounds it.

The Beauty of Sex

Sexual activity also is a way to express affection and love. In fact, in the biblical Song of Songs and in much secular literature, sexual intimacy is a model or analogy for other forms of love, including God's love for us.

Our sexual urges are a powerful sign of our longing to love and be loved. Communion with the beloved can be achieved in the sex act. The penis and vagina are the wonderful organs that allow this communion, the means of contact and intimacy.

The unity lost at birth can be rediscovered in sex. No more being alone: once again we can unite in a meaningful way with another human being. The sense of "us" that ended at birth is reestablished. Because sex embodies and expresses love, it is most *beautiful*.

The Joy of Sex

Sex is *fun*, perhaps the most pleasurable and exciting activity we adults enjoy. This is something that we have special difficulty admitting to our children—that sex is fun—as if children do not know, or as if the pleasure is wrong and we are ashamed. Or perhaps we fear that if we tell them it is fun, they will take that as permission to engage in sexual activity.

As with eating and sleeping, God made genital sexual activity pleasurable so we would want to do it. God made sex extra pleasurable so we would want to take the risk of caring, of fashioning a family, of loving. God uses the force and drive of sex to push us past the wall of shyness and loneliness and hesitation so that we dare to share ourselves with another.

Sex is a special way of expressing love physically. Of the same species as a handshake, a kiss and a hug, intercourse is more extreme because it involves our genitals, where a great profusion

4

of fine nerve endings are concentrated. This area is much more susceptible to pleasurable messages than other body parts. Sex is fun because it feels good and because it makes the partner feel good.

Good sex is adults at play. Play is a marvelous activity, a way of celebrating existence. One theologian said that next to love, the concept of play best expresses God's life and activity. God is play, at play with the universe, creating in joy and delight. In our sexual activity we are God's partners.

Sex is a microcosm of the art of living. It dissolves the tension between doing your own thing and loving your neighbor. It is good to do your own thing and enjoy your body. It also is good to love your neighbor, to pleasure your partner. In a larger frame this is the challenge of life: to love your neighbor as yourself. Good sex is a way of doing just that.

Sex Sold Short

Sex is fun, important, beautiful. What a letdown it is, then, to see sex presented in the media as carefree and uncommitted, as commercial, as a method of dominating. Such presentations sell sex short, accept sex as so much less than it can be.

Carefree and uncommitted sex has been described crudely as a "one-night stand" or worse. Frankly, that sounds sad, not even much fun. More realistically, since it is the nature of sex and love to promote attachment, that sounds hurtful. Imagine awakening yearning by a brief taste of intimacy and then attempting casually to shield against it.

Modern commercialism is even worse. Today sex is for sale. From soaps to porno films, gross and flashy sex is sold for cheap entertainment thrills. Even more, sex is added like a little sugar to sell everything else: cars, clothes, beer and toothpaste. That is like using Mozart to sell garden rakes—unutterably sad! Sex deserves a better press.

If that were not bad enough, sex also can be used to dominate and hurt. From the coldhearted person who "loves them and leaves them" to child pornography to sadistic cruelty, some modern sex is mixed with deception and violence. That is like mixing good wine with sewer water—a good way to spoil something fine.

Sex celebrates life and love. It is a big deal. Sex merits all the ceremony and all the drama that an inventive couple can devise. In no way is it casual or trivial. Sex should be fun, delightful, goofy, happy, provocative, silly—and yet easy to talk about and discuss. More, sex is very personal and intimate, terribly exciting, quite profound, the "main event."

A Positive Morality

The proper Christian attitude toward sex, stemming from the very nature of the generative act and of love, is positive. Sex is fun, important and beautiful: Christians must proclaim this good news in the face of the modern uncommitted and shabby treatment of sex. And parents must communicate these positive feelings to their children—not as a litany of don'ts and threats, but as something too marvelous to spoil by starting too soon and by engaging in sex outside the context of commitment and marriage.

The morality of sex derives from our nature as human beings. Therefore, families need no special and unique discipline for sex. Rather, sexual behavior (or misbehavior) should be included in the family's general approach to education and discipline.

What about the virtues of modesty and purity? The virtue of modesty can be presented from the point of view that the body and its functions are good and that modesty involves respect for the body. This is far different from saying the body is so shameful and its functions so naughty that it must not be displayed or even discussed.

The virtue of purity also can be presented positively, for purity and chastity involve the proper use of sex, not its non-use. As we shall see, occasions of sin are more likely to arise from curiosity and overstimulation than from an accurate knowledge of facts and functions.

Genital sex may be enjoyable and fun, but its morality is based on the fact that it is much more than fun. Sex is life-creating and sex is love-making. Because of this, sex demands commitment.

Sex demands an investment in the other person, the possible new life that waits for love to make it real as well as the beloved partner. All fairy tales end "And they lived happily ever after" because our instincts tell us that love is forever.

Commitment to another may be frightening. Any choice we make limits our other choices. Sex without commitment, however, is not the answer to the dilemma. Because we are human, uncommitted sex is a near impossibility. If things go well, attachment happens. Sex by its nature—by our nature—commits. People without commitment should refrain from sexual activity.

As any lovers will tell, commitment is not a burden but a joy. A lover will do anything, promise everything to the beloved. While fear of commitment may cause hesitation, the uncommitted life is not worth living.

Points to Consider

1) Although actual and truthful facts about sex are important, the attitudes you convey to your children are even more important. What attitudes do you have towards sex?

2) Attitudes color all our explanations and actions. Many adults have mixed-up or negative attitudes towards sex. How can you make your own attitudes more positive?

3) Why do many parents feel awkward discussing sex with their children? Think of ways to overcome or get around this awkwardness.

4) Try to develop a positive morality for sex. Why should people

be modest and chaste? You do not have to demean the joy and beauty of sex to raise moral youngsters.

Chapter Two

Beauty or Beast?

"Everything was fine till sex reared its ugly head." Thus one young lady described a difficult moment in a heretofore pleasant relationship. The "beast" of sex arrived to spoil the "beauty" of love.

Clearly, her boyfriend had physical feelings toward her which she did not reciprocate. Apparently he also was insensitive. But why blame sex? Blame the boy for trying to use her or for not being in touch with her wishes, but don't give sex an "ugly head."

Sexual urges wrongly have been identified with our nature as animals. The image of "the animal in us" conjures up fantasies of violence and uncontrolled passion reminiscent of Freud's id. Sex is highly emotional, something we think rational human beings should be able to control. Emotions are often seen as weakness, something we need to rise above and overcome.

A much better image than animal nature is the child in us. Children are playful, spontaneous, fun-loving and creative. A child letting go and running free is a much more positive and accurate picture of sex than an animal causing havoc. Sex awakens the child in us, not the beast.

Warnings Are Not Enough

Warnings about the dangers associated with sexual activity are not a substitute for information given in a positive and loving context. "We need more and better sex education. People have got to get in the habit of using condoms to prevent disease." These words by a prominent physician may be good advice, but they are not the essence of a good sex education. Sex education requires more than a list of prohibitions.

The thrust of much sex education is to prepare children to be careful copulators. We teach them how not to get pregnant and how not to get venereal disease. We secretly hope that if the warnings are dire enough, our young people will refrain from sexual activity altogether. We have been reluctant to prepare them to be good lovers, probably out of fear that if they really knew how fine sex was, they would start having intercourse early.

True morality comes from love, not from negation. Nevertheless, how many of us were introduced to the topic of sex by a list of don'ts? Today AIDS has become a terrifying concern, and fear of AIDS is used in an attempt to keep youngsters away from sex.

Authoritarians tend to use negative verbal control methods to train a proper response or scare someone into obedience. The pronouncements sound so right, but unfortunately they do not work very well. Saying something, commanding, even threatening severe consequences carry no guarantee that what the parent demands will happen. Even when the negative control methods work, it is at the high cost of depreciating the beauty of sex.

Keeping kids from premature sexual activity is surely a worthy goal. Demanding premarital chastity or threatening young people with the reality of dangerous diseases is not the best way to accomplish that goal. Threats are not an effective way to change behavior. How many TV ads focus on threats? They don't because that approach doesn't work well. TV ads are all positive, and they are rather effective at obtaining the desired result. Parents might learn something about good discipline from the advertising industry.

The Four Don'ts

Four don'ts head the list where sex is involved:

- Don't get pregnant.
- Don't get AIDS or VD.
- Don't do it unless you are married.
- Don't even talk about it.

Let's take a closer look at each *don't*.

Don't get pregnant. What a rotten idea to make pregnancy a threat and to make children the penalty for having sex! Children themselves, even when conceived out of wedlock, are beautiful. The parent or teacher who uses possible pregnancy as a threat or punishment to obtain compliance betrays an antichild bias. Children are a gift from God, not the price of misbehavior.

Don't get AIDS or VD. Some parents and teachers deliberately withhold information about how to prevent these dread diseases in the hope that ignorance will help keep children moral. I have even heard it said that sexually communicated diseases are the accounting God exacts from those who misbehave. Children ought not to be subjected to a pseudomorality that attempts to control sex by making it unnecessarily dangerous. Giving them appropriate information on how to avoid disease is not the same as giving them permission to have sex without marriage.

Certainly sexual intercourse should be saved for marriage. To make a case for that truth, however, one need not keep young people ignorant of acceptable means of disease prevention. There are better and more positive reasons for a strong morality and a Christian sex education. We do not need to threaten with the consequence of children or with preventable and treatable diseases. To do this is to denigrate God's greatest gift to us.

Don't do it unless you are married. Of all the don'ts, this is the least offensive. Of course it is wrong to have sex with someone

11

that is not married to you. One only wishes the morality were presented more positively, as: "When you have sex with your beloved spouse, love your partner tenderly and passionately and well."

One also wishes for some perspective on sin, for a morality that does not place sexual sins at the very top of the list. There are many other matters that appear far more hateful, such as cruelty and pollution and greed and war. For that matter, cheating on taxes is a sin that hurts everyone, but no one talks about that, perhaps because it is more likely to be a crime of the older adults who are doing the moralizing.

Don't even talk about it. Sex should not be discussed. The moralists who take this position like to quote Paul out of context when he said, "Immorality or any impurity...must not even be mentioned among you" (Ephesians 5:3). He was speaking in an exaggerated literary style to orgy-minded Romans, not to today's parents and teens. In a world which shouts its own jaded view of sex, we Christians are wrong to keep silent.

Silence Is Not Golden

Silence is not golden. Rather, it is a dangerous cop-out, leaving the field clear for the carefree and exploitative commercialism of TV, the crude messages on bathroom walls and the misinformation of older youngsters. The question is not whether a child will receive a sex education too soon, but what kind of sex education he or she will receive and who will provide it.

Silence about sex is itself an education. The implicit message is clear: Sexual matters are to be kept secret. Or, in so many unspoken parental words: "Don't talk to me about sex. I get embarrassed. It makes me uneasy. I'd rather pretend it's not there."

Unfortunately, parents with this philosophy only take themselves out of the picture. Even when children have a legitimate question or concern, they know better than to ask their parents. But do they remain totally uninformed about the issue? Hardly.

Curiosity is a powerful drive, even stronger than passion. Consider how many things dance through our minds within a short period of 60 seconds. Our minds are extremely active, hungry for sensation and information. Curiosity is the psychological counterpart to the physical sense of touch. It is vital to life.

More young people are led into premature sexual intercourse out of curiosity than out of passion. It is difficult to be passionate about something with which we have had no experience. Curiosity is therefore a major initial motivation for sexual activity. For this reason, it is of the utmost importance that parents satisfy a child's curiosity. An honest verbal explanation is surely preferable to premature blundering into sexual experience.

Our eagerness to learn, our imagination, our hunger for stimulation all drive us to discover. Almost universally, preschool boys and girls will peek at one another's genitals or even show them openly to one another. Bodies are on display in *Playboy* and similar magazines. Just because these opportunities are not available in our homes does not mean that our children will not see them.

More brazenly, TV displays couples making out and hopping into bed. Again, parents may forbid such viewing in their home, but there is no way to protect or shield a child from other children who have been thus educated and indoctrinated—or from bathroom walls with four-letter words and crude sexual rhymes.

Wouldn't it be better if the "good guys" got there first? Whatever parents have to say, even an awkward and stumbling admission of their discomfort, at least teaches the child sex is a subject which can be discussed with parents.

Points to Consider

1) What images come to mind when you hear the word *sex?* In our society many people have negative and crude associations to this word. Where do you think these negative images come from?

2) Emotions and passion are often seen as weaknesses which cause us to lose control. Yet our generally accepted life goals are emotional: to be happy or to love and be loved. Why then must our emotions take a back seat to reason? Can we trust our emotions? In what way?

3) Discuss this statement: A list of *don'ts* is not good discipline for any area.

4) Silence is not golden. Nor does parental silence guarantee that no sexual information and attitudes will be acquired. Is it possible totally to protect a child from any sexual information? Is this wise or desirable?

Chapter Three

Who? What? When?

In our awkwardness as parents and adults we can sometimes miss the obvious. We find it difficult to talk about sex with our children, so we mentally manufacture reasons to avoid the issue. Let's build some guidelines by asking three important questions: (1) Who should tell kids about sex? (2) What should kids be told? (3) When should particular facts be presented?

Who? The Parents

Who should give sex education to our children? That is an easy one to answer: The primary responsibility rests with the parents, not with schools or books or tapes. Ideally, sex education should not be something separate, a birds-and-bees talk, but should flow naturally as a part of the total family education about life and morality and love.

Why not the school? More and more, schools are assuming certain aspects of sex education. Schools provide information about anatomy and physiology in middle school or junior high, about methods of family planning and disease prevention in high school, and about sexual and lovemaking techniques in college. Nevertheless, public schools are expected to remain value-neutral. They cannot teach morals and say what is right and wrong. Church-supported schools teach morals, but they cannot provide the loving context for sex. Only the family can provide the natural, everyday education about sex that children need.

Parents are available, day in and day out; they are in the best position to answer questions *as they arise*. They are in the best position to keep sexual information within the larger context of life itself, to deal with sex not as a special topic, but as a part of everyday experience. Short informal exchanges are better than long talks. Parents have many more opportunities than school teachers or Church ministers to convey sexual information in a low-key and natural way.

Parents know their children best. Better than anyone else, they can individualize information to fit the needs of this child at this time. Parents are responsible for their children. They are not there to teach or preach for a year but to see their child into adulthood and beyond. Most of all, parents love their children. They care more deeply and personally than anyone about the total well-being of their child.

For all these reasons, parents have the primary responsibility and privilege to provide sex education for their children.

What? The Truth

What should be told? The truth. First of all, parents should use the proper terms. Right from the start *penis* and *vagina* should be used to name the genital organs. Private names each family has for the genital organs should be avoided.

Another aspect of telling the truth is that parents should never tell fables about sex. The stork and the cabbage patch are out. The truth can be told in general terms to very young children and details filled in later. For example, small children can be told that babies come from God. Later, they can learn that babies come from

God through their mother. Then they can learn that Father plants a seed in Mother. The original information should be something that can be built upon and enlarged.

There is more to the truth about sex than the genital act. Not only are there emotional, psychological and spiritual dimensions, but even on a physical level there is much more. We tend to view sex from a male point of view, much too narrowly.

If sex means all things connected with our gender, then we must also talk with children about menstruation and breastfeeding. Yes, boys, too, need to learn about menstruation, about how girls are "blessed with blood," as some societies so nicely put it. And girls need to hear about boys' sexual tensions and how a boy's desire for pleasure and creation can burst forth in nocturnal emissions or "wet dreams." Ignorance of these and other facts only whets curiosity and begets mistakes. Accurate information tends to calm a driving curiosity.

When? Early

When should sex education be given our children? Early. A major mistake many parents make is to wait too long—and thus allow knowledge from good sources to come too late, after the damage has been done.

The first rule is that sex education should be given naturally, as questions and opportunities arise. Births—of puppies or people—usually provide such an opportunity. Better early than late. Nevertheless, there are certain ages by which particular information should be complete.

Before they start school children should know where babies come from, how they get there and how they get out. If they do not know by this age, they will soon learn the answers from TV, older schoolmates and bathroom walls, and these answers will probably not be as good as the ones parents can provide, however awkward parents may feel.

One parent objected that early sex education was a mistake because the child did not need it yet. "I don't want my child to know anything about sex until he's ready."

This is like saying sailors should not read the hurricane manual until the first warning of a storm. They should read the manual while still in port, long before the information is desperately and immediately meaningful. Then, when the time comes to put safe procedures into operation, they feel reasonably comfortable and can do so more naturally. Sex education should be given long before the approaching storms of adolescence, when the information does not carry such a heavy meaning and can be dealt with more matter-of-factly.

At least one year before menstruation or nocturnal emission or by age 10, a child should possess more or less the full facts of life. If sex instruction is given only after the child menstruates or has a nocturnal emission, these experiences can be quite frightening. One 11-year-old girl had her first period while performing a cheerleading routine. When she saw the blood on her leg, she thought she was dying. A 13-year-old boy experiencing his first ejaculation feared he was coming apart. There is no reason to allow this type of trauma to happen through lack of preparation.

If a child does not ask questions about sex, parents should not think they have "lucked out." The child may sense the parents' awkwardness on the subject and may decide to look elsewhere for information. When a child is around age six, and certainly by age 10, parents must make opportunities to discuss sex if it does not arise in the normal course of daily living.

This is the important point: Parents should not wait on sex education while the child learns first facts and attitudes elsewhere. Rather, parents should talk about sex with their young child as opportunities arise, ideally before he or she begins school.

Points to Consider

1) Why is it so important for parents to talk about sex with their children? Why not leave this difficult topic to the schools?

2) Families have all kinds of private names for genitals. What is wrong with *penis* and *vagina?*

3) Discuss the statement: "Better too early than too late."

4) An important issue is whether accurate information allays curiosity or stimulates premature action. The author says that accurate information will be taken rather matter-of-factly by preadolescent children and is not as stimulating for them as it is for young adults. What do you think?

Chapter Four

A Firm Foundation

Preschool children are so young and so innocent. What a wonderful time to relate the beautiful story of how God takes us into a partnership in the continuing creation of life. He made man and woman incomplete, needing each other. Through sex they become one and their love for each other makes new life possible.

This incredible story should be what children learn first about sex and life and love. They should hear it when they are very young, while they are impressionable, before the world has a chance to make them callous and cynical.

Some parents object that small children are too young and innocent to be corrupted by knowledge of sex. Such an attitude implies that sex is evil, seducing us away from a more spiritual love. Such an attitude reflects the antisex bias of adults and is not protective of children at all. In fact, it leaves children vulnerable to all the world's abuse of sex.

Providing sexual information before it is vitally relevant helps keep the issue more natural and matter-of-fact. Delaying and hiding information gives sex unnecessary and unfortunate undertones. In their willingness to talk about it, parents communicate: "Sex is an OK thing."

Where Do Babies Come From?

Small children, like anyone else, are curious. They want to know where babies come from. "Babies come from inside their mommies, from under Mommy's heart, from Mommy's womb."

"You lived inside Mommy for a long time, almost a whole year, so close to Mommy's heart. I loved you as my new child. As you grew bigger, Mommy's tummy got bigger, too. Finally, when you were big enough, all ready to live and breathe and eat by yourself, you were born. You came out of Mommy and I was so happy to see what you looked like for the first time."

How does the baby get out? "There is a small opening between Mommy's legs called her vagina. Her vagina stretches to let the baby out. You were so big that stretching to let you out was hard work. That's why it is called labor. After you were born, Mommy's vagina closed up again. That is how you and everyone else were born. It is a beautiful story."

How Do They Get in There?

How do babies get inside their mothers? This is a legitimate question for a child to ask, yet one that is difficult for many parents to answer. Once we look past our own embarrassment, however, the truth is simple.

"You know how you love your teddy bear so much, and you hug him tight and love him until you practically wear his fur off? That is how Daddy loves Mommy and Mommy loves Daddy. And when Daddy hugs Mommy in a very special way, his penis enters into Mommy's vagina and a tiny seed passes from inside Daddy to inside Mommy. There it meets a tiny egg inside Mommy. With Daddy's seed and Mommy's egg and God's help, a baby is made. In the beginning the baby is so small that you can't even see it. But baby grows and grows until it gets big enough to be born."

The above is an abbreviated outline of how sexual information might be presented. This information usually satisfies children, and if properly given, rarely excites them with the urge to spread the "hot news" to the whole neighborhood.

One dad took advantage of an opportunity to tell his six-year-old son how babies are conceived. When the son heard about the penis entering the vagina, his response was a very predictable "Yuk!" A week later the same boy, while talking about kittens, asked his mother how babies got in and how they got out. When she reminded him that dad had just told him that last week, the boy answered: "Yes, but I forgot." This indicates that sexual information is not a vital matter in children so young—a major reason why it should be given so early.

Looking for Opportunities

Often children will not ask the "right" questions, or *any* questions about sex. Perhaps they sense that parents are reluctant to talk about it. Or perhaps they simply are not interested. Whatever the reason, parents need to look for opportunities to tell the story of life.

The story is best told naturally, in short segments, over a period of time. This is preferable to a one-time sit-down lecture by Dad or Mom. Single lectures are usually awkward and unnatural; they provide too much information for the child to digest all at once. Often they end with the parent asking: "Now, do you have any questions?" The child says no, and parent and child both are relieved that it is all over.

Opportunities abound. The cycle of life is all around us. One way for parents to get a discussion going is to see that the child witnesses the birth of an animal and to use that experience as a springboard for a natural conversation about sex.

Lucky is the child who gets to witness a birth! There is much a parent can say about how the little puppies get in, how they get out and what a beautiful thing life is. To see the mother dog lick off her young and then begin to feed them with her own body is a profound lesson about life. To embed sexuality into an atmosphere of wonder is the essence of a good sex education.

A pregnant woman, perhaps an aunt or an older sister, is another obvious starting point. "See Aunt Jessie, how big her tummy is? That's because she's carrying a brand-new, tiny baby in there. That's how I carried you with me before you were born." No need to carry this particular lesson further unless the child asks. The child has had a brief, on-the-spot, positive instruction in life and love.

The birth of a child is another golden opportunity. Who can help but be fascinated by a baby? What a fine time to make the association with sex! If the child is not overtly curious, the parent may want to frame a question or two. "Sometimes kids wonder where babies come from..." and then go on to give a brief answer. Parents must sometimes make their chances.

Growth in nature provides another beautiful context. "God's plan for life and love even works for corn and fruit and flowers." Parents can explain pollination, which leads naturally into the way humans exchange genes. The young child may not appear all that interested, but nevertheless it is important that he or she hear the story of life in such a natural and positive way.

When a small child observes a nude body of either sex, this, too, can be an opportunity for much worthwhile sexual information. "How come Mommy's got hair around her vagina and I don't?" is the parent's cue for a natural and normal description of some secondary sex characteristics and changes. "When you get older, some changes will take place in your body. You will grow hair around your vagina like Mommy, but other things will be changing inside your body, too. This is so you will be able to have babies like other big girls. It is a beautiful thing about being a girl."

Obviously, the child is getting a little more than she asked for, but parents who regard the question as a chance to share important information are taking advantage of an opportunity to give their daughter answers to questions she might not think to ask.

Even negatives can provide an opportunity. Suppose your small child inadvertently views a steamy scene on TV or is a party to some sexual activity among older youngsters. Parents can turn the lesson around by seizing the opportunity for some positive education. "You probably are wondering what that was all about. Well, God has this great plan about how life and babies get started when a man and a woman love each other sexually. You remember when I told you about that? Sometimes people are dumb; they use sex to hurt each other, or they try to take the pleasure without caring about babies or about the feelings of the other person. That is wrong because it spoils what God intended."

"Bad" words can provide parents with a similar opening. "Don't say that word. That's a dumb word for something beautiful, the special way that a man and a woman love each other and make babies. It's really called intercourse, but we also call it 'making love' because it can be a very loving thing. Did I ever tell you the story of how babies begin?"

Finally, if no opportunities occur and the child is ready to go off to school, parents may need to make their own entry. A parent might take the initiative through a comment such as: "You have probably wondered about babies, how they get started..." and then go on to explain, even if the child says he or she knows all about it. Better a few conversational comments on a number of occasions than one long formal lecture.

Show and Tell

Somewhere between three and six, a child will notice that both small and big people come in two varieties and will yield to curiosity. Children this age will experiment with their own bodies and peek at and explore the bodies of opposite-sex age-mates. Much of this goes on without parents ever becoming aware. Rather than be alarmed at this seemingly precocious fascination with bodies, parents need to see experimentation for what it is: a natural and normal and universal expression of curiosity. There is no need to be horrified. Instead, parents can treat it as a wonderful opportunity to begin sex education on a sound footing, to be there at the beginning with the proper information and attitudes.

The three- to six-year-old is more curious than sexy. Masturbation is a common activity at this age. Children play with their genitals initially out of curiosity and then because it feels good.

And so, when four-year-old Amy stands on the sidewalk with her hand inside the front of her panties, a matter-of-fact removal of the hand is sufficient. If Amy persists, Mother can continue to pull the hand up, perhaps adding: "We don't do that in public." Mother is wisely correcting behavior considered bad manners, yet she refrains from negative remarks about her daughter's genitals or sex.

Almost every child from ages three to six engages in a considerable amount of undressing, peeking and touching: "If you show me yours, I'll show you mine." This occurs in the tree house, under the covers, in the bathroom—anywhere children can find a certain measure of privacy from adults who might try to stop them. Children are learning. If adults get terribly upset about this normal curiosity, children may get the message that bodies and sex are bad.

Since much of this behavior stems from curiosity, early experimentation can often be decreased by appropriate parental sex instruction. If the "show and tell" is public, it can be discouraged simply and directly by telling the child, "Don't do that." No need to get wrought and indicate that something is frightfully wrong. Here parents are teaching good manners, not morality.

Sex education is best set in the context of physical affection. Modeling by parents is important. Children who experience touching and holding and physical comfort and who see their parents hold hands and hug and kiss will be more comfortable with later sexual feelings.

Good Touch/Bad Touch

The matter of child sexual abuse presents parents with a difficult dilemma. On the one hand, the sexual abuse of small children is much more common than we once imagined. So children need to be warned to avoid certain people and certain touches. On the other hand, it is a mistake to turn the child against all strangers and even against the natural pleasures of his or her own body.

Sexual abuse means the fondling of genitals or breasts with the intent to arouse, oral genital contact or sexual intercourse with a child. Children usually are abused by a male: a father, stepfather, brother, uncle or babysitter. One reason it goes unreported is because too frequently it is all in the family.

How do you explain sexual abuse to a young child who knows little or nothing about sex? You can't. The best protection is a positive education about the beauty and importance of God's gift of sexuality.

Unfortunately, sex education of the young is sometimes confined to a single prohibition: "Don't let anyone touch your private parts." That may be good advice, but it is not a sex education. Children need to learn about "bad touches," but they must be given a positive and more complete context.

Warnings against sexual abuse *must* be preceded by a positive and relatively complete sex education. This includes the proper names for genitals and other parts of the body, as well as a positive attitude and frame for this wonderful procedure of life and loving. Only then can the child understand why certain actions are abusive.

Here are some important things parents should know about sexual abuse:

1) It is not the end of the world. Unfortunate and wrong it surely is, but the child is not usually traumatized for life, nor will the experience necessarily spoil the child's later legitimate enjoyment of sex. A lot depends upon how the abuse is handled.

2) The local Welfare Department or abuse hotline will help you find good and understanding people who can help.

3) The offender is not necessarily a bad person but someone

who has done a bad thing and who can be rehabilitated. An offending family member may need to be separated from the family for a while and receive professional help but may return to the family at some point.

How should abuse be handled after reporting it? There are three issues which must be addressed with the child victim.

1) The child should be encouraged to talk freely about the incident or incidents as matter-of-factly as possible. This is no time for panic, which will only worsen the damage. Proper names for body parts should be used. Find out exactly what happened. This time to talk may last up to three months. If there is a police investigation, it should take place during this period. After this period, it is time to forget.

2) If the child has not already had a positive and rather complete sex education, he or she must have one now. Otherwise, what has happened will make no sense and be unnecessarily frightening.

3) The child must be assured that he or she has not done wrong, even if some pleasure was experienced. This can be a sensitive issue, but it is an important one to raise. Too many child victims feel great guilt because they may partially have enjoyed either the physical stimulation or the adult attention.

The possibility of sexual abuse is one more argument for sex education *before* any other influences become imperative. A major advantage to sex education during the preschool period is precisely that it is *not* critical yet. Sexuality can still be presented calmly and with lighthearted reverence. The facts themselves may be retained or forgotten, but the child will learn that sex is a proper subject for questions and discussion.

Points to Consider

1) "Where do babies come from?" "How do they get in there?" Practice answering these questions in an honest but reverent way so that you will feel more comfortable in talking with your child.

2) Go through a normal day and identify opportunities when you might point out to your child aspects of God's wonderful plan for continuing creation. Opportunities abound if you can become more alert to them.

3) Observe your child's curiosity. In a small child curiosity is a much stronger drive than sexual passion. Satisfying legitimate curiosity about sex will do much to put early experimenting to rest.

4) Nowhere does the good and bad side of human sexuality come into greater conflict than in the area of child sexual abuse. How can you maintain a positive attitude toward sex and still warn your child of potential dangers from abusive adults?

Chapter Five

Filling in the
Details

If basic sex education has been completed by the time the child starts school, then the next few years are a time to fill in the details. If sex education is not complete, then parents should take every opportunity to complete it quickly.

Beginning school means the appearance of a whole new set of outside influences. Less and less are parents the central source of attitudes and information. Now the teacher is viewed as an expert. The word of age-mates and older children is treated as gospel. TV's audiovisual power can make a strong impression. School, peers and TV may all have a lot to say about sex, not all of it good.

Anatomy and Physiology

Some major details to discuss during elementary school years are the names of all the parts of our generative systems and how they work for males and females. Anatomy is the parts list. Physiology tells how those parts work together to do what God intended.

Schools can do a good job of presenting the facts. Frankly, a listing of parts and their functions is not all that exciting. Parents may still be the ideal source for these facts, but they may have a hard time getting their child to sit still for the lesson.

There are many fine books, like *The Wonderful Story of How You Were Born*, that are filled with straight information and simple diagrams of body parts and functions. Parents might use such a book to refresh their own knowledge, or read the book together with their child. Anatomically complete dolls also may be helpful.

What are we talking about? Obviously, there is a lot more to sex organs than the penis and vagina.

A girl has an ovary on either side. This is where she makes her ova or eggs. When she reaches sexual maturity, one of her ovaries releases an ovum into the fallopian tube about once a month. The ovum heads down toward the womb, a cozy small pouch in the lower abdomen. If the ovum has met a sperm or seed from a male, it will probably fasten itself to the wall of her womb where it will be fed by a very rich blood mixture which the woman's body has prepared as a welcoming banquet for the new life. If not, the lonesome ovum will join with the blood and continue out through the cervix and flow out her vagina.

This is called menstruation, or the menstrual flow. It is a blessed activity because it means that the girl's body is doing its part in God's plan. During menstruation, to avoid staining her underwear, a girl will insert a tampon into her vagina or cover the vaginal opening with a sanitary napkin that absorbs the menstrual flow.

The adolescent boy's body undergoes similar preparations. Sperm are produced in the testicles carried in the scrotum. The sperm join with other fluids and make their way to and through the penis. Altogether, this fluid is called semen or seed. When there is a surplus of semen or when the boy becomes sexually aroused, extra blood will flow into his penis, making it stiff. This is called an erection. Sometimes this will happen during the night, and semen will discharge or ejaculate in spurts, with intense pleasure, usually accompanied by dreams of beautiful girls. This is called a "wet dream."

As the bodies of boys and girls prepare for their marvelous part in creating life, hair will begin to grow around the vagina and penis. Girls' breast size will increase, pleasing some girls and embarrassing others. Boys' penis size will also increase, with the same result: Some will feel manly and others awkward. The size of breasts has nothing to do with how much milk a new mother can produce. The size of the penis has nothing to do with how "masculine" a boy is.

Boys and girls become sexually aroused by kissing and caressing one another, especially by fondling the breasts, the penis and vagina. Corresponding to the boy's erection, a sexually excited girl's vagina will become moist so that the penis can enter easily.

What does all this mean to a boy or girl? It is not something to fear, and it would be silly to pretend it is not happening. Instead the child should give a big cheer: His or her body is working just right.

When the above information is presented in a matter-of-fact but reverent way, it is not all that stimulating. In fact, children are usually bored. That's OK. You just want them to understand that these facts are not lewd or vulgar and that there is no conspiracy of silence to keep the whole matter a state secret.

Obscene Language

The use of obscene words occurs from age three through senescence. In very young children they are probably an expression of curiosity. Parents would be wise to explain what the words mean and give the child the correct terms.

I remember the night when our first-grader asked politely at dinner: "Please pass the f---ing potatoes." We happened to have dinner guests. I nearly fell off my chair. As I later found out, he had heard that word on his way home from school. The children gave the impression it was a heavy word, so naturally he thought he ought to try it out at the dinner table. Our guests had all they could do to keep from laughing aloud.

Had I not been so surprised, it would have been a good opportunity to say something like: "Hey, that's a wrong word. We don't use that word around this house." Later on, I might have added: "It's a bad word for a beautiful thing, like when Daddy has sex with and loves Mommy very much and they might even start a baby." Meanwhile, I'd better pass the potatoes.

When older youngsters use such words, they are usually either expressing a cynical attitude toward sex or being mean to someone. Both issues are worth a brief parental response.

Our society is permeated with cynicism toward tenderness and affection. This cynicism is often reflected in sexual double meanings (accompanied by raucous laughter) or in outright crudeness. If the language is primarily lewd, parents can use the appearance of obscene talk as an opportunity to remind their child that sex is a beautiful activity.

If cruelty is involved, as in name-calling, parents might respond by saying: "Don't call anyone that. You are being mean." Instead of being upset by the superficial sexual content of the words, parents can react to the unkindness.

The wisest approach to bad language is to react with a brief and straight reprimand and then get on with the business at hand. Bad language is bad manners, like picking your nose or scratching your behind. Parents can teach their children not to use it without becoming overly upset and making it a moral crisis.

If the bad language persists, the first place to check is parental example. Many parents, especially fathers, have a loose or foul mouth of their own. Watch your own language.

Next, *ignore* the bad language. Some parents assume that ignoring means permitting, doing nothing. Ignoring is *not* doing nothing. Ignoring can be a very effective way of getting rid of certain disapproved behaviors. Remember the last time someone failed to respond to your "hello." If you are like most people, you probably felt bad all day. Behaviors do not continue without some attention or reward.

Finally, rather than responding to the bad words, reward your child for a clean mouth. I know one family that divided the day in half and gave "happy mouth" points worth some small reward for each half-day the child refrained from certain unpleasant words. The attention was focused on the good rather than the bad. The strategy worked.

Masturbation

Masturbation presents a difficult struggle for many youngsters, especially boys. On one side, there is a very strong urge to enjoy the intense pleasure that comes from stroking the penis or clitoris and to experience the ecstatic release of tension. On the other side, there is a strong prohibition against it because it turns something which should express committed love to selfish ends. The stronger the desire, the stronger some would make the prohibition.

Masturbation worries some parents greatly. They try everything they can to prevent masturbation, even infringing on the privacy of a child's bedroom, a serious parental mistake which gives too much attention to behavior best ignored.

In adolescence masturbation usually means continuing manipulation of the genitals to the point of sexual satisfaction. It calls for understanding, not condemnation. Although masturbation is *objectively* wrong, sinfulness also has a *subjective* dimension: the knowledge and freedom of the individual. Masturbation is very common among the immature: Statistics show that 95 percent of males and over 60 percent of females engage in such activity as adolescents.

Like the use of dirty words, masturbation is not a sign of eventual corruption and dissolution. Rather, it is a fairly normal attempt to explore the body—one that, with reasonable parental help, a child will outgrow.

A heavy-handed parental attempt to wipe out this activity now and forever may have unfortunate implications for the child's self-image. The child needs to know that his or her body and genitals are God's creation. They are not dirty, and the pleasures themselves are not sinful. On the other hand, parents need to know that they can tell a child to "stop it" without ruining the child's personality or future sex life.

For the most part, parents should leave the moral concern to their teen to work out with God. Checking up and constant lecturing on sin do not guarantee morality. Masturbation is an imperfect way to express ourselves sexually, but most of us grow constantly from the less than perfect to the more nearly perfect. Parents need to let that happen here.

TV or Not TV

TV provides a sex education and, in many cases, a poor one: sex without love, sex without children, sex without morals, crude and commercial sex. Children who already have a positive education in sexual facts and attitudes are much more apt to be immune to this message than those who have no other background.

Should parents try to monitor TV? Of course, but be careful. Remember that forbidding something may not be the best way to stop it. Forbidding certain TV shows may cause a child to sneak a bit, to spend a lot of time at the house of a friend whose parents are not so strict.

Parents also must remember that sex is not the only area where immorality is possible. In fact, there are worse things on TV than steamy sex: meaningless cruelty and violence, shows which teach and preach greed. To be consistent, parents should monitor all the problem areas on TV. Isn't this too much to do? Not really—if they take a more positive approach.

Instead of having a "forbidden programs" list, here is a four-point program to improve the quality of TV and to push the ever-present sex and violence and greed quietly to the back seat.

1) Parents should take inventory of their own TV-watching habits. *Parental example* is the most powerful way to influence a child's behavior. If parents watch "adult" movies or maintain a diet of *Rambo* and game shows, what can they expect of their children?

2) If parents are in doubt about the content or impact of a

certain TV program, they can sit down and *watch it together* with their child. Then, even if something troubling comes on the screen, it can become an opportunity for a potentially instructive and worthwhile discussion.

3) Parents can *limit daily TV time.* Two or three hours per day is a reasonable maximum. This will require children to seek other, less passive activities.

4) Parents can take a positive approach and help their children *select TV programs* of merit. Limiting TV time will necessitate their being more selective. Remember, however, that TV was meant to entertain as well as educate, so parents should not neglect programs that simply are fun.

TV is in itself a neutral factor. It can be used for ill or for good. As with sex, it is much wiser to focus on what is truly good and worthwhile rather than fight a constant defensive battle against all that is rotten.

Points to Consider

1) Can you talk comfortably and reverently with your child about sexual facts? If not, why not?

2) Ignoring is not doing nothing but a powerful disciplinary strategy for eliminating certain behaviors. If that is so, why are so many parents partial to lecturing?

3) How do you feel about masturbation? What do you think is the most effective way to respond to a child who masturbates?

4) How much time does your child spend watching TV? How much sex, greed and violence does he or she see? How can you monitor TV and make it an instrument for good?

Chapter Six

Adolescent Storms

Are early adolescents interested in sex? Of course! They are supposed to be. Sexual curiosity is normal at this age, only now it will receive a considerable boost from nature. If parents have talked openly about sex at an earlier age, the adolescent may continue to share some things, particularly factual questions, which parents need to answer accurately.

Most adolescents are reluctant to share their new feelings with adults. Even when parents have been accepting and open about sex, the adolescent picks up subtle messages in the home or in society. His or her new thoughts and feelings are not entirely acceptable, and the teen senses it. However permissive our society has become, boys still hide *Penthouse* and *Playboy* under their mattresses. Girls of 14 write explicit, passionate but unsigned letters, usually to older boys of 16 or 17 who have never looked twice in their direction.

Nude Magazines

Looking through nude magazines, watching adult television shows and going to X-rated movies are popular expressions of curiosity. How serious is such behavior? Much depends on the parent's view.

Some parents tolerate *Playboy* and attendance at adult movies as fairly harmless. These parents feel that forbidding such things only enhances their value and opens the way to lying and sneaking. As for these things being overstimulating, I doubt it. Nothing—no magazine, no mere picture—can compete with fantasy. As one priest-journalist remarked: "Nothing is so prurient as the mind of a 15-year-old boy."

In fact, a good case can be made for deliberately ignoring such behavior. Better to focus on the positive aspects of sex, the pleasure, the importance and the beauty, than to give "adult" films or magazines time or attention which might paradoxically encourage them.

A danger in making a concerted effort to get rid of these magazines is that parental attention will keep them in the spotlight. The youngsters may simply hide them or look at them elsewhere. I, for one, wish rather to focus not on the tawdriness but on the bright and loving side of sex.

Other parents feel strongly that such portrayals must be expressly forbidden. Parents *can* forbid, but at the same time they should avoid condemning sex itself. It is important to give a complete message: "I don't want you reading these magazines *because* I feel they give a demeaning and vulgar view of sex. Sex is beautiful, it is attractive and it is fun. These magazines cheapen sex and women and men." Such parents forbid in a more positive way. They express their own views and feelings; they condemn the vulgarization of sex but not sex itself.

The simple solution if you don't want such magazines around the house is to throw them out. Explain that such portrayals are irreverent, and leave it at that.

Discipline

Wise parents have provided a basic education in sex long before adolescence. Now they may feel they need to hold the line against the twin assault of teenage hormones and a society with rather loose sexual morals. They are right. Parental lectures are not likely to be effective in influencing teen behavior. Frankly, teens do not listen much to what parents say. They look more to peers for counsel and support. Group discussions about sex with teens are possible and good, but even there it is best to let teens talk and share their own thoughts and feelings rather than try to "straighten them out."

Sometimes schools and Churches approach the subject of sex through a process called "values clarification." This sounds like a good idea, but every time I have listened in, the adults were trying to get the teens to come around to the adult way of thinking and to indoctrinate them. The adults are "clarifying" adult values for the teens, not helping the teens clarify their own values. Teens usually react to this by tuning out; it does not work. Teens need to be heard before they can be moved.

The best way to pass on values about sex is through parental example. If the teens witness a loving physical relationship between their parents, if sex is discussed in the home with playful reverence, if sex is not coupled with crudity and dominance, then teens will have an excellent context in which to fit their beginning understanding of sex. If, on the other hand, the parents are mean to each other, physically distant, perhaps even in the process of divorcing, then it will be difficult to present sex in a loving context.

While not exactly sex education, practical discipline assumes great importance during the teen years. Teens may not pay much attention to what parents say, but parents need to be quite firm about what rules they set, particularly about curfew and about preventing situations which are an invitation to sexual intercourse. A discussion about proper values and behavior with a hormone-riddled teen is not as likely to be effective as getting that teen home on time, away from alcohol and drugs, out of parked cars and into constructive activities.

Parents can never control sexual behavior with certainty; they cannot be aware of their teenager's whereabouts at all times. Parents, however, can limit chances for sexual experiences by setting and enforcing a curfew. A teen who is home by a certain time will get into less trouble. Observing curfew is behavior parents *can* control.

In addition, parents can *somewhat* control where the teenager goes when he or she leaves home. If Ann is going to a slumber party Friday night at Lisa's, Mother might well call Lisa's mother just to be sure that the facts Ann gave are accurate. If Tim is going to a big party at a friend's house, Dad is wise to make sure that Tim's parents know about the party and will be home that night. If Terri is going to babysit very late on a Saturday night, Mother might call the parents who hired her just to be sure that she does indeed have a late-night babysitting job.

Such checking is justified. Parents have the right to know where their teenager is. If the teen says, "You don't trust me," parents can pass it off lightly: "I'm concerned about you out there in the big bad world." Or they might answer more seriously, "I'm concerned about you, and I want to be sure that I know where you are." Only a very naive parent would say: "I trust my teenagers completely and would never check up on them."

Saying No: Abstinence

Sex makes babies. That is one of its two main functions. The other is making love. If sex is not likely to be either fruitful or loving, then it should not happen. A teen should say no.

Saying no is not always easy. The teenager's glands and would-be partner are both saying yes, yes, yes! So how can kids say no?

They need first to have confidence in themselves. They need to be strong enough to stand against the crowd and against their own rising desire. The teen that can do this has a mind of his or her own.

Unfortunately, obedience to parental rules does not always encourage a mind that can stand its own ground. It may create a follower mentality and, when obedience to parental rules breaks down, the teen follows his or her peers.

To stand up for one's own beliefs, a teen must be spunky, even ornery. Parents need to encourage their teens even in mistakes, supporting their right to make their own choices.

In the matter of saying no to premarital sex, parents might encourage their sons and daughters to stand up for what they believe, to dare to be different: "Your body is your own. You may feel pressured to go 'all the way.' But you know there are other considerations: your feelings of tenderness and love, learning how to be close friends. Putting on a condom may protect you from pregnancy or disease, but what can you put on that will protect your heart and soul and that of your partner? You need more time to grow so that you can experience all there is to sex and not just 'get laid' for the fun of it. Until you are ready in every way, pray for the strength to say no."

Only fools, however, put all their trust in good intentions, no matter how sincere. Parents also can help their teens by minimizing or eliminating situations where sex is possible or likely. Allow teens some privacy for physical affection in your own home, where intercourse is much less likely to result. Let them have friends over for video films or parties. But don't leave teens home alone. Try to keep them out of parked cars.

Sex happens, but it is more apt to happen when couples are alone, drinking and without fear of being interrupted. Saying no means avoiding these situations.

Being Careful: Contraception

Teenage pregnancy is a serious concern for parents, perhaps more than for the carefree teen. Some parents mistakenly believe that teaching children about natural family planning and contraception is the same as telling them that unmarried sex is OK. That is not true. There are many compelling and understandable reasons to advance against premarital sex. Presenting positive arguments for chastity is much wiser and safer than keeping youngsters in ignorance of the means to prevent pregnancy.

Adolescents have the need and right to know about both moral and immoral solutions to the problem of an unwanted pregnancy. Keeping our young people *ignorant* is not a wise way to try to keep them *moral.* Yet the dilemma of presenting information about means we consider immoral is both touchy and difficult.

First of all, our society, unlike our Church, is democratic. Contraception is both a legal and a practical option. Whether we parents like it or not, our young people really can choose contraception and even abortion. If we refuse to discuss these matters, then our young people will go elsewhere to someone who will. The parent who is open and honest about the possible options and the means to these options is more likely to have teens who will bring home the hard problems.

It helps to remember that the divine Parent gives us a wide variety of choices. God does not force us or hide information about immoral choices. All choices are open to us in God's creation.

Much more critical than whether these options are discussed is *how* they are discussed. Yes, the teen should have information about contraception and abortion. More importantly, this information should be presented in the context of family and religious values. Family may be the only place where young people can hear about contraception and abortion within the frame of a sound, healthy and positive understanding of lovemaking and its fittingness in marriage.

This does not mean parents are giving their children a license to have sexual intercourse. It does mean that parents must talk and work with their growing children about the whole problem of morality. They should be teaching their children how to become moral beings, how to arrive at responsible moral decisions.

This is different from blind obedience. For too long we have viewed morality as a set of rules, a set of answers. Our children are about to become adults. They should learn how to ask moral questions, how to weigh moral decisions for themselves.

Should teenage girls be on the "pill"? If they are already sexually active and are going to continue to be, no matter what the parents say, then they need to know the facts, including how various contraceptive methods work. They also need to know that the estrogen in the pill may interfere with their development, that some pills are abortifacients, that condoms don't always work.

If a young person asks for contraceptives, that is a rather clear indication that he or she is or is about to become sexually active. Lack of proper information from parents is not an effective or wise way to stop them. Rather, parents may see this as an opportunity to provide the information within the context of a healthy and positive sex education with a positive emphasis on purity. If the young person still chooses to use contraceptives, parents need to accept his or her right to do so. Human freedom—even to do wrong—is part of God's plan for creation.

Here is a very brief review of artificial methods of birth control. These all prevent the sperm and egg from meeting and are therefore judged immoral by the teaching of the Church.

1) The *condom* or "rubber" comes like a rolled-up balloon. The male rolls it down over his penis to catch the sperm during intercourse.

2) The *pill* is an artificial female hormone which a woman takes regularly by mouth to tell her body not to produce any eggs. It may have unpredictable and harmful developmental effects in the immature female.

3) The *diaphragm* is a soft rubber cup or cap which fits snugly over the cervix, the entrance to a woman's uterus or womb. It works like a bathtub plug to keep the sperm from reaching the egg.

4) *Creams or jellies* are strong chemical agents inserted into the vagina before intercourse to kill or immobilize sperm. They are most effective when used carefully and with a diaphragm.

5) The *intrauterine device* (IUD) is an object inserted in the uterus which prevents any fertilized egg from attaching itself to the uterine wall. This causes abortion: The fertilized egg is then washed out in the menstrual flow. IUDs are used less and less

because they have proven sometimes to be dangerous to women.

6) A *vaginal sponge* is a small sponge which is placed in the vagina after having been soaked in sperm-killing chemicals.

7) A *tubal ligation* is a surgical procedure for the female in which the fallopian tubes are tied or cut, preventing any eggs from reaching the uterus. It is not usually reversible.

8) A *vasectomy* is a similar surgical procedure in the male where the tube that carries his sperm is cut and the sperm run into a dead end. Like the tubal ligation, the vasectomy is usually permanent and irreversible.

The only method of regulating births approved by Church authority, *natural family planning*, includes two methods. The *rhythm method* limits sexual intercourse to that time of month when a woman is not likely to conceive. Its effective use requires that a woman have regular periods and that she keep careful track of the days between. The other method is called the *symptomo-thermal* or *ovulation method*. It enables a woman to attend carefully to her body temperature and to the mucous discharges from her vagina so she can tell when ovulation occurs. Both methods call for planning, being careful and periodic abstinence during fertile days.

There is more to the question of pregnancy prevention than method. Children are our tomorrow. They have the potential to open our hearts farther than we thought possible. On the other hand, there are definitely times when a child would strain the health or well-being of a family. A couple may want to make love without making a baby. Parents need to help their teens understand that this choice is vital and important and to help them understand the logic behind Church teaching.

Some condom ads refer to "safe sex," meaning safe from pregnancy and/or disease. Young people need to learn that uncommitted sex is never "safe," that just being careful may protect you from becoming a responsible and committed person or learning what a free and giving person you can be. Sexual intercourse begets intimacy; liking turns to love and "safe" sex can cost a broken heart.

Respecting Life: Abortion and Suicide

What do you do when your son announces his girl is pregnant or your daughter tells you that she is pregnant and wants an abortion? This may be the toughest problem of all because there are no easy solutions. The fact that your child has confided in you and asked for your help indicates that you have done a good job of childrearing so far. Now is no time for a parental lecture. You and your youngster need to talk.

Teenage pregnancy does not mean that you have been a bad parent. Sex does sometimes happen too soon, and sometimes babies happen. Parenting is coping and helping your children deal with life's problems as they arise. You now have a big one.

Your daughter's pregnancy emancipates her. She is now biologically an adult and legally entitled to make her own choice. Parents can help by spelling out four acceptable options: marriage; raising the child as a single parent; letting parents raise and/or adopt the child; and releasing the child for adoption.

Parents must be careful not to *impose* their advice. The choice belongs to the young persons, to both of the parents-to-be. Parents can shed some light and wisdom on the issue by helping the young people consider finances and schooling and how the baby will affect their life or lives. But those directly involved must be involved in the ultimate decision.

Should they marry? If they were already planning marriage, this may be the simplest solution. If not, a marriage forced by pregnancy has a very poor chance of survival. One mistake is enough. Listen to them. Help them to talk through the possibility of marriage.

What about adoption? Adoption may be the best choice for the unborn child, but it is not always easy for the family to accept. Some parents would require their daughter to keep and raise the baby as a "punishment" for what she has done. That is very wrong because it does not consider what is best for the coming child and the young mother.

Open adoption is a choice selected by many families. Parents adopt their son's or daughter's baby, but the son or daughter is obviously allowed to have continuing contact with the child after the adoption is legally completed. Open adoptions can be arranged with friends as well. This has the advantage of permitting the young parents to feel they are not abandoning their baby and, at the same time, assuring that the child will be raised by responsible and mature adults.

The girl can raise her child as a single parent. While difficult, this is not impossible. I have known very young mothers who do a marvelous job with their babies. Parents should be very clear with their daughters, however, about what they as grandparents will and will not do. Keeping the baby and then giving it to Grandpa and Grandma to raise while daughter grows up is not really being a mother. In this case it would be better for the grandparents to adopt the baby. One important matter to clarify in any discussion is the practical and concrete description of what parenting entails and who is going to do it.

There are two other very real possibilities which, while not morally good, are frighteningly available: abortion and suicide. Both choices often occur to pregnant unmarried teens. The first may be suggested by peers. The second may originate deep inside her mind, fueled by fear that "my parents will kill me when they find out."

Some parents make the mistake of dismissing abortion and suicide as unthinkable. Immoral as these choices may be, there is overwhelming evidence that they are disturbingly real and not at all unthinkable. If your daughter is thinking about them, you need to discuss them with her—and you need to do so with as open a mind as possible, without passing judgment on her.

Suicide talk may sometimes be a bid for attention or sympathy. Suicide also may seem the only way out of a situation that appears hopeless. Parents may be tempted to dismiss such talk as self-serving or unlikely. This is a mistake. The option of death must be addressed.

The likelihood of suicide can be lessened in two ways. First, an exploration of all the other options should help reduce the apparent hopelessness. The youngster must feel free to discuss even choices of which parents do not approve. Second, the parents can respond with warmth and understanding to the suicide talk: "I'm sure you feel terrified. This is a very difficult moment for you." This is surely a much better response than, "Don't talk like that!"

All the options must be open to discussion. The failure to discuss abortion because the parent refuses to consider it only deprives the parent of any input. It may be unthinkable to the parent but, unfortunately, it is surely not undoable. If parents won't discuss it, daughter may talk it over with her friends and leave parents out. Peers have sometimes collected money to pay for an abortion the parents never know about.

Abortion is not an easy way out. Many young people have had abortions without much forethought, only at a later time to be overwhelmed with guilt at what they have done—frequently during a subsequent, wanted pregnancy.

Abortionists tell their patients never to look at the material vacuumed or cut out from the womb because it is too upsetting. Of course it is upsetting! All of us have very strong instincts against harming anything that looks helpless or human. Most of us would have difficulty killing a small puppy or kitten. Reverence for life means trusting in this basic instinct to preserve and protect what lives.

Unfortunately, now may not be the time to share all these thoughts with your daughter. If it sounds too much like a lecture, she may not listen. This is one more strong reason why a complete sex education, including a discussion of abortion, should be accomplished *before* it is necessary.

Parents clearly have moral values of their own, and they have a right to make these known. A parent might tell his or her daughter: "Although I will respect your feelings and decision, you also must respect mine. That is my grandchild in your womb. I cannot abide abortion, and I cannot say it's all right or help you obtain an abortion."

Parents, however, should stop short of threatening to disown their daughter. They might add: "If you go ahead and get an abortion on your own, though I disagree, I will respect your right to make a choice, and I will continue to love you." This may be hard for some parents to say. Nevertheless, it is the way God treats all of us, and we parents must strive to match God's unconditional love.

AIDS and Other Dangerous Diseases

One subject we would rather avoid because it is unpleasant and not "nice" to talk about is sexually transmitted diseases (STDs). Knowledge about STDs is not license to have "safe" sex, nor is ignorance of STDs and their causes a wise strategy to scare a young person into being moral. Young people have the need and right to know about STDs: cause, prevention and treatment.

The STDs may be caused by viruses, bacteria or other organisms that thrive in moist, warm places, such as the mouth, genitals or rectum. Thus they can be transmitted through vaginal, anal or oral sexual contact but are not likely to be passed on through contact with toilet seats, doorknobs or drinking cups. Deep kissing, tongue-to-tongue, is a possible means of infection, however.

Briefly, there are seven common STDs. Teens need to learn about them. All are preventable, and all except AIDS and herpes are curable.

Syphilis occurs in three stages. In the first stage an open sore (chancre) develops, usually on the penis or inside the vagina. A rash or swelling in the groin may develop as well. These symptoms may develop from 10 to 90 days after contact. The sores last two to five weeks and then disappear, but the disease does not go away. The second stage is marked by moist, flat warts appearing around the genitals, accompanied by fever, sore throat and headache. This may begin any time up to six months following stage one. The third stage of syphilis affects the spinal cord and brain and may not develop for many years. If treated in stage one, syphilis is curable through antibiotics. A physician can make a correct diagnosis.

Gonorrhea ("clap" or "drip") causes a yellow or white discharge from the genitals that begins five to 14 days after sexual contact. The World Health Organization lists gonorrhea as second in frequency only to the common cold among infectious diseases. Penicillin is the best treatment.

In *herpes, type II,* small blisters which burn and itch and cause tenderness may appear on the genitals, thighs or buttocks. Although the symptoms may disappear in one to three weeks, the virus does not, and most people will have recurrences throughout their lives. Active herpes can be passed on to a baby during childbirth. For this reason, a Caesarian section may be recommended. There is no known cure for herpes.

Venereal warts (Papilloma virus) are usually painless, although they may cause itching. There is growing concern that this virus is connected with cancer. The warts can be chemically or electrically removed.

Pubic lice ("crabs") are parasites that cling to the pubic hair and bite the skin to suck the blood, causing severe itching. Treatment includes an external cream or lotion or wash that can be obtained from a pharmacy.

Chlamydia (Pelvic inflammatory disease or PID) is a general infection of the pelvic organs signaled by pain, vaginal discharge, fever and/or prolonged menstrual bleeding. An antibiotic is usually effective against chlamydia.

AIDS (acquired immunodeficiency syndrome) is the most feared of the STDs and legitimately so: It is fatal, and there is no known cure. First reported in 1981, AIDS is a disease caused by a virus that can damage the brain and affect the body's ability to fight off illness. AIDS itself doesn't kill, but it allows other serious diseases to enter the body and kill. Fatigue, long-lasting infections and swollen glands are common first symptoms, but these also are common to other diseases. When in doubt, see a physician. The only sure way to diagnose AIDS is a blood test.

Can you touch someone who has AIDS? Yes, you can. There

is no evidence that AIDS is spread through casual contact, such as shaking hands, coughing, sneezing, social kissing or sharing swimming pools, bed linen, eating utensils, cups and so on. There is no reason to avoid ordinary social contact.

How is the AIDS virus spread? Mostly in three ways: through anal sexual contact, through the use of contaminated needles and through contaminated blood supplies. Today blood products are routinely tested for the AIDS virus so that a person is now extremely unlikely to get AIDS from an infected blood transfusion.

Can you get AIDS from having normal sexual relations with an infected partner? Yes, but this is still rather uncommon (estimated at under 10 percent of reported cases by 1991). You cannot tell if your partner has AIDS. Most people who are infected look and feel healthy.

The safest way to avoid any STD also is the moral way: to say no to sex with anyone except a spouse and to be mutually faithful.

If one has sex in a moment of passion, it will help somewhat (but not much) to wash the genitals carefully as soon as reason returns. A condom offers limited protection against getting an infection from a partner who may be at risk. A person who has any reason to suspect any of the STDs, especially AIDS, should see a physician immediately for the appropriate testing.

All the STDs, especially AIDS, carry a strong public stigma. Since the great majority of AIDS victims to date have been either homosexuals or intravenous drug users, many persons have taken the attitude that AIDS is the victim's own fault and that he or she therefore deserves no sympathy.

Such condemnation leads to the isolation of the AIDS sufferer. Friends and acquaintances desert the ill person. Some fear contagion; others feel they cannot do anything for the victim and wish to avoid feeling helpless. Still others prefer not to be reminded of their own mortality. Social support, so necessary for any terminally ill person, is hard to find.

All through history some people have seen certain diseases as God's punishment for sin. AIDS is seen as God's newest avenging angel. This is both unfortunate and un-Christian. AIDS claims many totally innocent victims. Even with those who appear to be at some fault, this is not God's way of punishing guilt.

Some parents have been shattered to learn that their young adult child has AIDS. Today's best information indicates that they can safely do the loving thing: bring the patient home.

The fact of suffering and death should elicit compassion in us. Those who work with the dying know that the message of approaching death is to live what one has left of life to the fullest, to treasure the todays, not mourn the tomorrows. Parents who tend AIDS patients often tell their child all those things they never had the time or the courage to say; they go places, do things that they and their child would like to do together.

Sexuality is a gift from God to make life and love grow. If sometimes certain dread diseases are communicated through sex, that is not cause to be critical and judgmental but reason for concern and compassion. In this spirit of love parents need to pass on knowledge about sexually transmitted diseases and AIDS.

Homosexuality

What shall we tell our teenage children about homosexuality? We need to tell them the truth. Ignorance breeds prejudice and fear and meanness. Sooner or later our teens will meet gay persons, and they should know better than to use such names as *queer, homo, lesbo, faggot, fairy* or *dyke.*

The first thing we need to do is distinguish between homosexuality itself and homosexual *activity* (oral or anal intercourse). Homosexuality in its simplest form is a preference to exchange physical affection with members of one's own gender. In other words it's an attraction to members of one's own sex. As with heterosexuality, it need not involve genital activity.

Homosexuality is common enough. An estimated four to 10 percent of the population prefer sexual contact with members of their own sex. They have the same physically affectionate feelings towards same-sex members that the rest of us have toward members of the opposite sex.

Being homosexual is not an either-or matter. Sexual preference is more like a continuum. Most adults fall somewhere near the middle but closer to the heterosexual limit. For example, many married adults enjoy sexual relations with their spouses but at the same time will express physical affection in the form of a big hug or a handshake with a member of their own sex. Some predominantly heterosexual adults will occasionally even experience a "crush" on another person of their own sex. This is quite common. Homosexuality and heterosexuality are not so much categories as they are matters of degree.

Many experts suspect that homosexuals are born that way. Others believe that sexual preferences are irreversible by age four or five, certainly by adolescence. If not inborn, homosexuality appears to be part of constitutional development and not the result of faulty learning or poor parenting. Homosexuality is not a habit but a powerful drive, one not likely to be altered.

Homosexual inclination is one thing; homosexual behavior another. *Being* homosexual is not a moral issue; we do not will or choose our sexual orientation. Catholic teaching condemns homosexual activity. We can judge behavior; only God can judge persons. Homosexuals deserve the same respect we give any person—and, in light of the AIDS plague, they deserve additional help and compassion.

Gays are not bad people; one's sexual preference does not make a good or bad person. There are many homosexuals who are beautiful people and who have accomplished much. They are not "sissies" or "butches" but come in all personality types. Gays are not necessarily genitally sexually active. In sum, they are people like everyone else, with the same hopes and fears but with an unalterably different sexual orientation, one that both they and the rest of us must learn to live with.

Teens need to know that an occasional homosexual urge or action does not make someone gay. We all are likely to have such temporary inclinations. Nor does one become a homosexual by having gay friends. It is not contagious. Should a gay friend make an "advance," teens can offer thanks for the affections while indicating they are not so inclined.

Some sex differences are physiological. Men, due to hormonal differences, generally are more active and aggressive; women are more physically maternal. But, although male and female *gender* is inborn, *roles* are not. The woman's role is learned, like any other behavior. Many traits considered feminine are attractive in either sex: gentleness, intuitiveness, artistic temperament, a quiet disposition. They should be encouraged in both boys and girls. They are not evidence of homosexuality. Besides, homosexuality is probably a genetic or constitutional matter, and parents are not likely to either cause or change it.

More than in other areas of sex education, with homosexuality parents may need to take the initiative. They cannot expect a question: "What about homosexuality, Dad?" More likely they will overhear some slur against gays. Parents need to seize such an opportunity to present the facts and to share their feelings and Christian values.

The issue is much larger than sexuality. It goes right to the core of being a Christian. Sexuality is morally neutral, but charity is not. We Christians have a moral mandate to love our neighbor, especially when our neighbor is needy and even when our neighbor appears undeserving.

Further, Jesus told his followers not to judge. Even when our neighbor appears morally at fault, unless that fault harms another person, the matter rests between our neighbor and God. Rarely if ever does personal criticism change behavior. It is more apt simply to be an expression of our mean self-righteousness.

Homosexuals have a special burden to bear in our society. As sexual beings ourselves, we need not approve or adopt their sexual preferences, much less their sexual activity, but we have no reason to blame or mock them. They are different, and differences are OK. They need our companionship and esteem as persons—as do all our neighbors.

Broken Hearts

The most common problem of all for teens is a broken heart. It is a lucky parent whose teen confides the pain of rejection. There is no hurt like the loss of a first love.

Boy-girl love is infused with sexuality, whether there is sexual activity or not. This makes such relationships heated and wonderfully urgent and, when one party breaks the relationship, it seems like the end of the world.

What can a parent do? First of all, listen. Don't be too quick to reassure. Let your teen spill out the grief and the emptiness and the anger.

Then share. Remember your own heartbreaks and share them. Tell about the times you thought your own life was over because someone did not return your love.

Finally, remind your teen that true love is an attitude, not an object. It is a trait of the lover and does not demand return. The important issue is that your teen continue to reach out and be a loving person, even though in this relationship, he or she feels hurt and rejected. Your teen may need your support and help to be able to trust and love again.

True love is like sexual activity: It has a selfish side wherein one takes personal delight, but its basic thrust is outward, to explode and expand. Genital sex leads to procreation, the incarnation of the love between two people. Love reaches beyond the person, beyond the loving couple. That is why all the world loves a lover: because a person truly in love has a smile for everyone.

Love surely has its stumbles, its setbacks, its broken hearts. An understanding parent can do much to maintain a teen's courage to love a world that sometimes does not love back.

Points to Consider

1) Sexual misbehavior is not the only sin. Why do some parents seem so much more concerned about genital behavior than about greed or violence or drugs?

2) Do you think parents should ever provide contraceptives to their teenage sons or daughters? If so, under what circumstances?

3) When parents take a firm stand on certain issues, teens know better than to talk with their parents about that matter. They know they'll get a lecture. How can parents share their own values with teens and still communicate that *all* issues are open for discussion?

4) Many people have strong negative feelings towards homosexuals. How can parents deal with their own negative feelings before sharing with their teens?

Chapter Seven

When Children Become Adults

What is left to teach the young adult child about sex? We've talked about the beauty and the abuse, the passion and the problems. Hasn't everything been covered? What do those who are about to marry still need to learn?

They need to learn how to be good lovers. Ideally, parents might take some time with their grown children to share any bedroom talents. Fathers might pass on lovemaking techniques they have learned to their sons and likewise, mothers to their daughters.

If sex is a good thing—and it is a *very* good thing—then it is surely worth doing well. Insofar as lovemaking is a skill, the lovers-to-be should learn all they can about the ways and means. Unfortunately, truly good sex has been a well-kept secret in our culture, as if it were wrong to have fun and to pleasure our companion to the edge of ecstasy. In any case, parents in our culture do not easily share sexual techniques with their children. If parents find it difficult to share their "best moves," perhaps they can at least communicate that sex should be fun and frolicsome. Good sex is adults at play.

Stag or hen parties during the week before the wedding are a ritual way our culture introduces the about-to-be-married to the joys of sex. These parties, however, tend to be high on alcohol and crude jokes and low on useful sexual information. Perhaps they better serve a simpler purpose: to say good-bye to an unmarried friend.

Making Love Right

Much of today's instruction for nearly-weds comes from books and classes. I would look for a book that combined playfulness and reverence with lots of examples of lovemaking possibilities. *The Joy of Sex* by Alex Comfort (Fireside, 1972) is such a book.

Pre-Cana classes offered by the Catholic Church may be another example of good instruction. In my pre-Cana classes 30 years ago, however, I learned about sex from a physician who showed us his medical slides. They were a bit grim. The lecture was serious and heavy, and sex certainly did not sound like much fun. I truly wondered whether lovemaking was something I would want to do very often.

I since have attended other classes for the engaged where the part on sex is given by an older married couple. The facts are there, and even the playfulness, but they often have an attitude about sex which does not fit the more preoccupied excitement of the engaged.

The best presentations about how to be good lovers come from young marrieds, couples who have been married three to five years. That is long enough to become good at loving and still young enough to be eager and excited.

Education about any subject should be concerned with teaching how to do it well. Why should sex be any different? To say that sex comes naturally, that the best sex instruction will be the education the two neophytes provide for each other in learning together, is another cop-out. Such an excuse reflects our difficulty in discussing sex as a playful and pleasurable activity.

There are many possible sexual positions which young

marrieds can present nicely through stories with reverent humor. Times and places can be varied, from the bedroom to the bathtub. Lovemaking can be enhanced with candles and wine, with lingerie, with body oils and massage. I have heard young married couples present all these possibilities for good loving lightheartedly and yet with great respect.

Good sex means consideration for your partner, knowing how to pleasure your partner, how to give him or her the best time possible. Since life has its rough moments, there are times when a good loving will be very important. The ability to pleasure your partner well does not come naturally. Much new knowledge of anatomy and physiology can help all of us become better lovers. A major part of good sex education for young people should teach how to pleasure your partner and love well.

Dealing With Adult Kids

The transition from child to adult should be marked by a change in the relationship between parents and child. Instruction and rules take a back seat and are replaced by support for the person. Grown children are best regarded as friends.

Few parents in our culture see their grown children as friends. Considerable tension often exists between parents and their young adult children. The popular press describes differences in values, behavior and life-style as the generation gap. One suspects that the thinking and behavior of older children cause the parents guilt, disappointment and a sense of failure.

Parents sometimes feel frustrated and guilty because, as the child grows, they try to control him or her in essentially the same ways they controlled the young child but with less and less success. Such control is inappropriate for adult children. Rather, when adults relate to each other in mutually supportive ways, we call that friendship.

Young adults frequently vacillate between wanting more freedom and fearing the responsibility of adulthood. When a child asks parents for advice, the urge to comply is almost too tempting.

What parent would not be flattered, eager to direct the child along the wise path which the parent sees as best?

Decision-making, however, is part of becoming an adult. Rather than giving advice, parents must help the young adult to make the decision, to explore and define the alternatives which exist, perhaps by writing down the pros and cons of each. The parent who takes over the decision-making process creates a no-win situation. The child cannot take credit for whatever good comes from the decision because the decision was not his or hers. And the parent can be blamed for any wrong that results because it was a parental decision. Even more important, the young adult child loses an opportunity to grow.

This same parental restraint applies just as surely to moral decisions. Human beings can learn and grow from mistakes, even mistakes in moral matters. Parents must respect their adult children's rights to make their own moral choices.

For example, Sue is dating a divorced man and wants to bring him home to have dinner and meet the family. Her family is distressed. They feel angry because they cannot understand or tolerate her behavior and frustrated because they cannot do much about it. Parents often blame themselves and wonder where they have failed. Whatever the personal disappointment, parents would do well to recall that adults are personally responsible for the values, decisions and life-style they choose. Parents are not responsible for the behavior and decisions of their adult children.

At the same time, parents need not give their unqualified support to everything their adult offspring do. How should parents react when their children choose a behavior or a life-style which is incompatible with their own values? Using the friendship guideline, parents might ask themselves: How would I react if my best friend, my neighbor, my boss behaved this way? In general we should treat our adult children at least as well as we treat our other friends.

Some parents believe: "If we can't approve it, we must condemn it." They often find themselves at a loss when their adult child moves in with a person of the opposite sex. Shocked and hurt at seeing their values so rudely rejected, they seek ways to get the young adult back to a Christian way of living.

Unfortunately, changing the behavior of an adult is beyond parents' power. Instead, they can consider the options which really are open to them:

1) They can refuse to have any social contact with either partner until and unless they change their behavior. There is real danger in that position. They lose a child now by their own choice and, in the event of a later marriage, they may not be able to reestablish a relationship.

Parents who judge that living together out of wedlock constitutes such un-Christian behavior that they must refuse to associate with someone who acts this way might ask themselves if they apply the same standard to other un-Christian behaviors.

2) They can accept their own child but reject the partner. They can say, "You are welcome in our house, but he or she is not." In effect, they are saying, "My child is OK. This situation is all the other person's fault." This position hardly seems fair. It takes two to make a live-in couple.

3) They can accept both partners as adults, not approving the choice they have made, but recognizing that the choice is the couple's, not their own.

There is a difference between acceptance and approval. Acceptance means recognizing that God himself gives all of us the right to make moral decisions and, no matter what we choose, he keeps right on loving us. God is a very good psychologist who knows how best to reach people: You love and support them even when they appear to be wrong.

Parents can, however, propose some "house rules" for grown children. House rules can be parents' way of expressing their own moral values in practical terms. They tell what parents will and will not tolerate in their own home.

The first rule might be: "In my house you may not sleep in the same room with someone to whom you are not married." They might add: "I love you and respect you. Please show me the same respect. I can't let you have unmarried sex in my house because I feel that would be cooperating with something I believe is wrong."

The parent above makes an important distinction between the person of the child and his or her chosen life-style. Parents may abhor the life-style of their grown children. They need not collaborate or cooperate with what they hold is wrong. But parents still must keep on loving.

With adult children it is no longer effective to mandate behavior and to punish misdeeds. They are often unreceptive to parental counsel or advice. Like the mother of St. Augustine, however, parents can continue to rejoice at their legitimate successes, to help their offspring up again when they stumble, to love them, to be there.

That, after all, is what family and love—and sex—are all about.

Points to Consider

1) Do you feel your own sex education prepared you to be a good lover? How do you want your children to approach their wedding nights?

2) How do people you know deal with their adult children's moral choices when they do not approve? Are their methods effective or hurtful?

3) What people have influenced your behavior, even caused you to reconsider and change it? How did they achieve such influence?

Afterword

The best sex education is accurate information set in a context of family love and integrity. Before a child begins school, he or she should have an outline of the story of life. Long before first menstruation or nocturnal emission, children should possess the complete facts in some detail. If opportunities to present this information do not occur naturally, then parents should look for or make opportunities.

Parents will inevitably communicate attitudes and values about sex in the way they cope with the usual questions and problems that arise as children grow and develop.

Sex is fun. Sex is beautiful. Sex is holy and important. These are the positive attitudes that must underlie the family story of God's most wondrous gift.